DEDICATION

To my beloved family, whose unwavering support and encouragement have been my anchor throughout this writing journey. Your love fuels my passion, and I dedicate this book to each of you.

To the readers who embark on this exploration, may you find inspiration, insight, and moments of connection within these chapters. This book is dedicated to the pursuit of knowledge and the shared journey towards growth and understanding.

With gratitude and love,

Dr. pete

How Not to Suffer: Uncover the Practices Clinically Proven to Enhance Your Sexual Health

Dr. pete

CONTENTS

ACKNOWLEDGMENTS

Writing a book is a collaborative effort that involves the support, encouragement, and expertise of many individuals. As I express my gratitude, I would like to extend my heartfelt thanks to those who played pivotal roles in the creation of "How Not to Suffer"

Firstly, I would like to thank my family for their unwavering support throughout this writing journey. Your encouragement and understanding during the late nights and weekends devoted to this project are deeply appreciated.

I extend my gratitude to the healthcare professionals, researchers, and experts whose work and insights have contributed to the foundation of the book. Your dedication to advancing knowledge in the field of sexual health has been a beacon for this project.

To my friends and colleagues who offered encouragement, understanding, and occasional distractions during moments of writer's block – thank you. Your support has been a source of inspiration.

Special thanks to the readers who embark on this journey with "How Not to Suffer." Your curiosity and commitment to long-term intimate wellness are the driving force behind this work.

Lastly, a profound thank you to all those unnamed individuals who, directly or indirectly, have influenced and shaped my understanding of the topics covered in this book. Your collective contributions have enriched the content and depth of "How Not to Suffer."

Lastly, a profound thank you to all those unnamed individuals who, directly or indirectly, have influenced and shaped my understanding of the topics covered in this book. Your collective contributions have enriched the content and depth of "How Not to Suffer."

This book is a reflection of the collaborative spirit that drives progress, and I am deeply grateful to each person who has been a part of this venture.

INTRODUCTION

Welcome to a journey of empowerment and discovery – a guide crafted to transform your understanding of sexual health and well-being. In a world where intimate wellness is often discussed in hushed tones, "How Not to Suffer: Uncover the Practices Clinically Proven to Enhance Your Sexual Health" invites you to break free from the shackles of silence and embark on a path toward a more fulfilling and vibrant intimate life.

As a society, we frequently navigate the complexities of health, yet the intricacies of sexual well-being often remain veiled in mystery. This book seeks to unravel the science behind sexual health, bridging the gap between conventional wisdom and evidence-based practices. This guide endeavors to revolutionize the conversation around sexual health.

Understanding the Foundations: The Interplay of Nutrition, Lifestyle, and Sexual Health

In this introductory chapter, we lay the groundwork for a comprehensive exploration of sexual health. Delve into the interconnected web of nutrition, lifestyle choices, and their profound impact on your intimate well-being. By understanding the foundations, you'll gain the knowledge needed to make informed decisions that can positively influence your sexual health journey.

Join us as we navigate the multifaceted aspects of sexual well-being, exploring topics ranging from hormonal balance and stress management to fertility and overall lifestyle choices. By the end of this journey, you'll be equipped with practical insights and evidence-backed strategies to enhance your sexual health and embrace a life of vitality and fulfillment.

Embark on this transformative odyssey with an open mind and a willingness to explore the intricate dance between science and sensuality. "How Not to Suffer" is not just a book; it is an invitation to reclaim control over your intimate well-being, fostering a life rich in passion, connection, and enduring satisfaction. Let the journey begin.

PART I: UNVEILING THE FACTORS IMPACTING SEXUAL HEALTH

Embark with us on an illuminating journey into the foundational section of "How Not to Suffer." Within these pages, we set forth on a compelling and comprehensive exploration that aims to unravel the intricate tapestry of factors influencing sexual health. Part I serves as a rich landscape, inviting readers to delve deep into the multifaceted dimensions of hormonal balance, stress management, and fertility—key components that intricately shape the contours of one's intimate well-being.

Our intention is to not merely skim the surface but to plunge into the depths of understanding, laying bare the complex interplay between physiological processes and the delicate nuances of human connection. These chapters serve as portals into realms where hormones orchestrate the symphony of desire, stress weaves its threads into the fabric of intimacy, and fertility stands as a beacon guiding the way to a thriving reproductive well-being.

1 HORMONAL HARMONY: NAVIGATING THE PATH TO A BALANCED LIBIDO

In the realm of sexual well-being, hormonal balance plays a pivotal role in shaping the experiences of desire and satisfaction. Let's embark on a journey through Chapter 1, where we unravel the science of hormones in a practical and reader-friendly manner, providing actionable insights for cultivating a balanced and fulfilling intimate life.

Understanding the Hormonal Symphony:

Hormones are like the conductors of a symphony, directing the ebb and flow of desire within our bodies. To make this concept more approachable, think of hormones as messengers that transmit signals between different parts of your body, influencing everything from mood to energy levels, and, of course, sexual desire. Key players in this symphony include testosterone, estrogen, and progesterone.

Exploring the hormonal symphony is not about diving into complex scientific jargon but about gaining a simple appreciation for the incredible dance happening within your body. As we navigate this symphony, we'll shed light on how these hormones work together to create the melody of a balanced libido.

The Impact of Hormonal Imbalances:

Imagine hormonal balance as the sweet spot where desire and satisfaction harmonize. However, various factors – be it stress, lifestyle choices, or underlying health conditions – can throw this harmony off balance, resulting in hormonal imbalances. These imbalances may manifest as fluctuations in mood, energy levels, and, importantly, libido.

Practical Insight: Recognizing the Signs - Pay attention to changes in energy, mood swings, and fluctuations in sexual desire. These can be indicators of potential hormonal imbalances that may need attention.

Strategies for Hormonal Health:

Now, let's get practical. Nurturing hormonal health doesn't require complex rituals; it's about incorporating simple habits into your daily life. Consider the following:

1. Nutrient-Rich Diet: Opt for a balanced diet rich in essential nutrients that support hormonal health. Include foods like whole grains, fruits, vegetables, and healthy fats. These provide the building blocks your body needs for optimal hormone production.

2. Regular Exercise: Physical activity is a natural mood booster and plays a crucial role in hormonal balance. Incorporate exercises you enjoy into your routine, whether it's brisk walks, yoga, or dancing. Consistency is key.

3. Stress Management: Chronic pressure can wreak havoc on hormonal balance. Practice stress-reducing activities such as meditation, deep breathing exercises, or engaging in hobbies you love. These simple practices can have a profound impact on your hormonal well-being.

4. Adequate Sleep: Quality sleep is a cornerstone of hormonal health. Ensure you get sufficient and restful sleep each night, as it directly influences hormone regulation.

Holistic Perspectives on Hormonal Well-Being:

Hormonal well-being extends beyond the physical aspects and incorporates emotional and mental dimensions. Here are practical insights to consider:

1. Emotional Well-Being: Cultivate emotional health by fostering positive relationships, expressing emotions, and seeking support when needed. Emotional well-being contributes to a more balanced hormonal environment.

2. Mindful Living: Incorporate mindfulness into your daily life. Engage in activities that bring you joy, practice gratitude, and be present in the moment. This not only reduces stress but positively impacts hormonal balance.

3. Lifestyle Choices: Make conscious choices in your lifestyle. Limit alcohol intake, keep away from smoking, and hold a wholesome weight. These lifestyle factors contribute significantly to hormonal health.

Embracing Hormonal Changes:

Life is a journey, and so is hormonal health. Hormonal dynamics change across different stages, from adolescence through adulthood to the golden years. Understanding and embracing these changes is key to fostering a healthy and enduring libido.

Practical Tip: Communicate- If you're in a relationship, open communication about hormonal changes can strengthen the bond with your partner. Understanding and supporting each other through different phases can enhance intimacy.

In wrapping up this practical exploration of hormonal harmony, remember that small, consistent changes can lead to significant improvements in your intimate well-being. As you integrate these practical tips into your life, you'll find yourself not only navigating the hormonal symphony but dancing to a melody of balance and satisfaction. The journey to a balanced libido starts with simple, actionable steps, and Chapter 1 is your guide to making these steps a part of your everyday life.

2 STRESS AND INTIMACY: STRATEGIES FOR A TRANQUIL CONNECTION

Imagine a bustling city, filled with the honking of horns, the rush of people, and the constant demands of daily life. This city represents the stress that often infiltrates our lives, affecting not only our well-being but also the intimate connections we hold dear. In Chapter 2, let's explore the profound relationship between stress and intimacy, weaving in practical strategies and a touch of storytelling to guide you on the path to a more tranquil connection.

The City of Stress:

Meet Alex and Jamie, a couple navigating the bustling city of stress. Juggling work, family, and countless responsibilities, they often found themselves entangled in the chaotic rush, leaving little room for moments of tranquility and connection. As stress became a constant companion, their intimate life began to feel the strain.

Mapping Stress:

Stress isn't just a mental burden; it infiltrates every aspect of our being. It influences our physical health, emotional well-being, and, significantly, our intimate relationships. As we navigate the city of stress, it's essential to map out its impact on our lives, especially on the connections we hold dear.

Practical Insight: The Stress Map - Take a moment to reflect on the sources of stress in your life. Identify areas where stress may be affecting your intimate connections, and consider how these stressors manifest in your daily interactions.

Creating Tranquil Oases:

In the midst of stress, Alex and Jamie decided to create tranquil oases within their bustling city. These were moments of reprieve, where stress took a back seat, and the focus shifted to nurturing their connection.

Mindful Moments:

The first strategy our couple employed was introducing mindful moments into their routine. Whether it was sharing a cup of tea in the evening or taking a short walk together, these simple practices allowed them to be present in the moment, fostering a sense of tranquility and connection.

Practical Insight: Mindful Micro-Moments - Incorporate small, mindful practices into your day. It could be a brief pause to take a few deep breaths, savoring a quiet moment together, or even sharing a heartfelt conversation.

Digital Detox:

Recognizing the impact of constant digital connectivity on their stress levels, Alex and Jamie decided to embark on a digital detox journey. They set aside specific times to disconnect from screens, creating space for genuine, uninterrupted connections.

Stress-Reducing Activities:

In their quest for tranquility, our couple explored various stress-reducing activities. From practicing yoga to engaging in creative pursuits, they discovered that dedicating time to activities they enjoyed alleviated stress and brought them closer together.

Practical Insight: Discover Your Stress-Busters - Identify activities that bring you joy and relaxation. It could be anything from gardening to listening to music. Incorporate those stress-busting sports into your routine.

Communication as a Bridge:

One key lesson Alex and Jamie learned was the importance of communication as a bridge over the tumultuous river of stress. By openly expressing their feelings and concerns, they found mutual understanding, strengthening their connection in the face of life's challenges.

As you navigate the city of stress in your own life, consider implementing these practical strategies. Create your tranquil oases, embrace mindful moments, and let communication be the bridge that fosters a deeper connection with your partner. In the chaos of life, may you discover moments of tranquility that breathe life into your intimate connections.

3 FERTILITY FITNESS: ENHANCING REPRODUCTIVE WELL-BEING

Let's embark on a journey through Chapter 3, where we'll explore the fascinating landscape of fertility. Picture a garden filled with diverse flowers, each representing the unique aspects of reproductive well-being. This chapter will guide you through practical insights, weaving in storytelling to make the journey toward fertility fitness more accessible and engaging.

The Garden of Fertility:

Meet Sarah and Chris, a couple strolling through the vibrant garden of fertility. Each flower represents an aspect of reproductive well-being, and as they navigate the garden, they discover the keys to enhancing their fertility.

Understanding the Fertile Soil:

Just like a garden needs fertile soil to flourish, reproductive health thrives in an environment of overall well-being. The soil represents various factors such as a balanced diet, regular exercise, and emotional wellness that contribute to fertile ground for fertility.

Practical Insight: Planting Seeds of Nutrition - Consider incorporating fertility-friendly foods into your diet, such as leafy greens, whole grains, and foods rich in antioxidants. Think of it as planting seeds for a healthy garden of fertility.

Sunshine of Exercise:

In the garden, sunlight is essential for growth. Similarly, regular exercise provides the necessary sunshine for reproductive well-being. Sarah and Chris discovered that incorporating physical activity into their routine not only improved their overall health but also positively influenced their fertility.

Hydration, the Nourishing Rain:

Just as rain nourishes the garden, staying well-hydrated is vital for reproductive health. Sarah and Chris made it a habit to drink plenty of water, recognizing its role in supporting fertility and overall wellness.

Practical Insight: Sip to Fertility - Keep a water bottle handy throughout the day as a reminder to stay hydrated. It's a simple yet impactful way to nourish your reproductive garden.

Weeding Out Stress:

In any garden, unwanted weeds can hinder growth. For Sarah and Chris, stress acted as those unwanted weeds in their fertility garden. By incorporating stress-reducing practices like meditation and deep breathing, they created an environment conducive to reproductive well-being.

Restful Sleep, the Gardener's Reprieve:

Just as a gardener needs rest to tend to the garden, quality sleep is crucial for reproductive health. Sarah and Chris prioritized a restful night's sleep, recognizing its role in hormonal balance and overall fertility.

Practical Insight: Cultivate a Sleep Routine - Create a calming bedtime routine to signal to your body that it's time to unwind. This can consist of sports like reading, mild stretching, or practising rest techniques.

Blooms of Emotional Connection:

The most beautiful flowers in the garden represent the emotional connection between Sarah and Chris. Nurturing their emotional bond not only brought joy to their relationship but also positively influenced their fertility journey.

As you navigate your own garden of fertility, consider planting seeds of nutrition, bathing in the sunshine of exercise, and weeding out stress to create a fertile environment. Hydrate your garden with the nourishing rain of self-care, and let the blooms of emotional connection flourish. May your journey toward fertility fitness be as vibrant and fruitful as the garden you tend to with care.

PART II: NUTRITION AND LIFESTYLE SOLUTIONS FOR A THRIVING SEX LIFE

Welcome to the heart of your transformative journey – a section meticulously crafted to unravel the secrets of a more vibrant and fulfilling sex life through the realms of nutrition and lifestyle choices. Imagine this section as a tapestry, each thread representing a practical, evidence-backed strategy that has the potential to revolutionize your approach to intimate well-being.

4 THE POWER OF NUTRIENT-RICH FOODS: A SENSUAL FEAST FOR SEXUAL VITALITY

In the realm of intimacy, imagine your journey unfolding as a sensorial adventure, akin to a carefully curated feast for both body and soul. As we step into Chapter 4, we delve into the transformative power of nutrient-rich foods – the ingredients that can elevate not only your culinary experiences but also the vitality of your intimate life.

The Culinary Odyssey Begins:

Meet Emma and Alex, a couple embarking on a culinary odyssey to explore the aphrodisiacal wonders of nutrient-rich foods. Their journey began not as a prescription but as an exploration of flavors that resonated with their shared passion for well-being and connection.

Storytelling Element: Picture a cozy evening where Emma and Alex decide to transform their usual dinner routine into a sensual feast. Consider sharing a personal experience of a special meal that holds sentimental value for you.

A Symphony of Flavors:

The world of nutrient-rich foods is a symphony of flavors, each note contributing to the orchestration of vitality. From oysters known for their zinc content to the richness of dark chocolate with its antioxidant properties, Emma and Alex discovered that the key to a sensual feast lies in the diversity of nutrients.

Practical Insight: Crafting Your Sensual Feast - Consider experimenting with a variety of nutrient-rich foods known for their aphrodisiac properties. From avocados to strawberries, let your meals become a celebration of sensual nourishment.

Zinc: The Elixir of Desire:

Zinc, often heralded as the elixir of desire, became a focal point in Emma and Alex's culinary exploration. Foods rich in zinc, such as pumpkin seeds, lentils, and seafood, took center stage in their meals, influencing not only their taste buds but also their intimate vitality.

Practical Insight: Zinc-Infused Delights - Incorporate zinc-rich foods into your meals. From a delightful pumpkin seed salad to a seafood extravaganza, infuse your menu with these nutrient-packed delights.

Omega-3 Fatty Acids: The Dance of Passion:

Imagine the dance of passion ignited by the presence of omega-3 fatty acids. Foods like fatty fish, flaxseeds, and walnuts became the protagonists in Emma and Alex's culinary tale, contributing to the harmony of their intimate well-being.

Storytelling Element: Envision a shared moment where the flavors of omega-3 rich foods become a part of your shared experience. Share a personal story of discovering the delights of these nutrient-packed ingredients.

Antioxidants: The Spark of Connection:

Antioxidants, the spark of connection, found their way into Emma and Alex's culinary repertoire. Vibrant berries, dark chocolate, and colorful vegetables became not just a visual feast but an infusion of vitality that sparked connection and rejuvenation.

Practical Insight: Vibrant Infusions - Introduce antioxidant-rich foods into your meals. Experiment with a berry-infused dessert or a colorful vegetable stir-fry to add a burst of vibrancy to your sensual feast.

Culinary Exploration as Connection:

The culinary exploration for Emma and Alex became more than just a journey through flavors; it became a shared experience that deepened their connection. The act of crafting meals together, experimenting with new recipes, and savoring the results became a ritual that nourished not only their bodies but also their intimate bond.

Storytelling Element: Share a personal story of a culinary exploration that became a memorable experience for you and your partner. Highlight the connection forged through the act of creating and enjoying meals together.

As you step into the realm of nutrient-rich foods, let this chapter be an invitation to embark on your own culinary odyssey. Craft your sensual feast, infuse your meals with the power of nutrients, and let the flavors become a celebration of intimate vitality. This is not just about what you eat; it's about creating moments of connection and passion through the shared experience of a sensual culinary journey. The feast awaits, and the flavors are yours to explore.

5 BEYOND THE PLATE: LIFESTYLE CHOICES THAT IGNITE INTIMACY

Imagine your life as a canvas, and each brushstroke represents a lifestyle choice that contributes to the masterpiece of your intimate well-being. In Chapter 5, we journey beyond the plate, exploring the vast landscape of lifestyle choices that have the potential to kindle the flames of passion and foster a deeper connection.

The Metropolis of Life:

Visualize your life as a bustling metropolis, filled with various avenues and thoroughfares. In this dynamic cityscape, we follow the story of Mia and Liam, a couple navigating the bustling metropolis of life, where daily stressors and responsibilities threatened the tranquility of their intimate connection.

Storytelling Element: Paint a picture of Mia and Liam's daily life, showcasing the challenges and joys they experience in the vibrant metropolis of their shared existence.

Stress Management as Urban Planning:

Just as a well-designed city prioritizes green spaces for relaxation, Mia and Liam realized the importance of incorporating stress management techniques into their daily routine. They discovered that practices like meditation, deep breathing, and mindful walks acted as green havens amidst the concrete jungle of stress.

Practical Insight: Create Your Urban Retreat - Identify stress-relief practices that resonate with you, whether it's meditation, yoga, or simply taking a few moments for deep breaths. Transform your daily routine into a sanctuary for stress management.

Shared Adventures as Communal Streets:

The city of life became more vibrant for Mia and Liam as they explored shared adventures. Engaging in activities like hiking, dancing, or even cooking together transformed their relationship into a communal street, fostering shared joy and connection.

Storytelling Element: Share a personal experience where engaging in a shared adventure strengthened your connection with your partner. Highlight the sense of camaraderie and joy these activities brought into your relationship.

Digital Detox: Clearing Traffic Jams in Communication:

Recognizing the digital traffic jams that often hindered communication, Mia and Liam decided to embark on a digital detox journey. They designated specific times to disconnect from screens, creating clear communication lanes and fostering genuine, uninterrupted connections.

Practical Insight: Establish Communication Lanes - Set aside dedicated times for a digital detox. Whether it's during meals, evenings, or weekends, creating communication lanes free from digital distractions can enhance the quality of your connection.

Quality Sleep as Urban Renewal:

In the city of life, quality sleep became a form of urban renewal for Mia and Liam. They prioritized creating a restful environment, ensuring that the night offered a time for restoration and rejuvenation.

Storytelling Element: Reflect on how prioritizing quality sleep positively impacted your overall well-being and intimacy. Share a moment where a good night's sleep became a catalyst for connection.

Emotional Connection: The Heartbeat of the City:

The heartbeat of the city is the emotional connection between its inhabitants. Mia and Liam discovered that open communication, vulnerability, and small gestures of affection were the essential beats that resonated in the heart of their relationship.

Practical Insight: Strengthening Heartbeat Connections - Cultivate open communication, express vulnerability, and incorporate small gestures of affection into your daily interactions. These emotional connections form the heartbeat of your intimate city.

As you navigate the bustling metropolis of your own life, consider the urban planning of stress management, explore the communal streets of shared adventures, and clear communication lanes through digital detox. Prioritize the urban renewal of quality sleep and nurture the emotional connections that form the heartbeat of your intimate city. Let Chapter 5 be a guide to infusing vitality and connection into the urban landscape of your shared existence. The journey continues, and the vibrant city of intimacy awaits your exploration.

PART III: A HOLISTIC APPROACH TO SEXUAL HEALTH

Welcome to the section that delves into a holistic approach to sexual health. In these chapters, we'll explore practical and evidence-based strategies that encompass various facets of well-being, promoting a balanced and fulfilling intimate life.

6 MIND-BODY CONNECTION: CULTIVATING EMOTIONAL WELL-BEING FOR ENHANCED INTIMACY

Welcome to a pivotal exploration of the mind-body connection and its profound influence on emotional well-being, a cornerstone for enriched intimacy. In this chapter, we unravel the intricate relationship between our emotional state and the quality of our intimate experiences, providing both understanding and practical strategies for fostering emotional wellness.

1. Understanding Emotional Well-Being:

Embark on a journey into the intricate landscape of emotions and their impact on sexual health. Recognize the nuanced ways in which feelings such as stress, joy, anxiety, and contentment can influence desire, arousal, and overall satisfaction in intimate relationships. By grasping the interconnected nature of emotions and sexuality, you lay the foundation for a holistic approach to well-being.

2. Practical Strategies for Emotional Wellness:

Navigate the realm of practical strategies designed to cultivate and maintain emotional well-being. From mindfulness practices to evidence-backed stress management techniques, explore actionable steps that empower you to build emotional resilience. Discover the transformative power of activities such as meditation, deep breathing exercises, and journaling, which can contribute to a positive emotional state, setting the stage for more fulfilling intimate connections.

Practical Insight: Integrate short mindfulness exercises into your daily routine. Whether it's a brief moment of focused breathing or a mindful walk, these micro-practices can accumulate, fostering emotional well-being over time.

3. Enhancing Communication in Intimate Relationships:

Communication forms the bedrock of emotional connection. Dive into effective communication strategies that facilitate understanding, vulnerability, and a deeper emotional bond between partners. Learn to express desires, concerns, and feelings in a way that promotes open dialogue and fosters intimacy. Communication is not merely verbal; delve into the significance of non-verbal cues and active listening to enhance emotional connection in your relationship.

Practical Insight: Set aside dedicated time for intentional and open communication with your partner. Create a safe space where both of you can express your thoughts and emotions without judgment, strengthening your emotional connection.

As you navigate the terrain of the mind-body connection in this chapter, remember that emotional well-being is an ongoing journey. By incorporating these practical strategies into your life, you not only enhance the quality of your intimate experiences but also contribute to your overall sense of fulfillment and happiness.

7 FITNESS FOR FULFILLMENT: EXERCISE STRATEGIES TO SUPPORT SEXUAL HEALTH

Embark on a journey into the world where physical fitness intertwines with sexual well-being. This chapter explores the dynamic relationship between exercise and intimate health, shedding light on how various forms of physical activity can contribute to heightened arousal, improved stamina, and an overall more satisfying intimate life.

1. The Link Between Exercise and Libido:

Unlock the secrets of how exercise influences libido and sexual function. Delve into the physiological responses that occur during physical activity, such as increased blood flow, the release of endorphins, and improved cardiovascular health. Understand how these factors collectively contribute to heightened sexual desire and a more robust intimate experience.

Practical Insight: Experiment with different types of exercise to identify what resonates with you and your partner. Whether it's aerobic activities like running or cycling, strength training, or yoga, find the balance that enhances your overall well-being.

2. Tailoring Your Fitness Routine for Sexual Health:

Discover how to customize your fitness routine to specifically target aspects of sexual health. From cardiovascular workouts that improve circulation to strength training that enhances muscle tone and flexibility, learn how intentional exercise can positively impact intimate experiences.

Practical Insight: Consider incorporating interval training into your routine. Short bursts of intense exercise followed by periods of rest can boost cardiovascular fitness, contributing to improved stamina and energy levels.

3. Yoga and Sensuality:

Explore the fusion of yoga and sensuality as a holistic approach to sexual well-being. Uncover specific yoga poses and practices that promote flexibility, mindfulness, and heightened body awareness. From enhancing the mind-body connection to reducing stress, discover the multifaceted benefits that yoga brings to intimate health.

Practical Insight: Integrate partner yoga into your routine, fostering a sense of connection and trust. Shared yoga experiences can deepen the bond between partners, contributing to a more satisfying and harmonious intimate life.

As you delve into the relationship between fitness and sexual health, remember that the key is finding activities that bring joy and align with your preferences. By incorporating intentional physical activity into your life, you not only enhance your overall health but also contribute to a more vibrant and fulfilling intimate experience.

8 SLEEP AND SENSUALITY: MAXIMIZING REST FOR OPTIMAL INTIMATE WELL-BEING

Welcome to a crucial exploration of the often underestimated connection between quality sleep and sensuality. In this chapter, we uncover the profound impact that sleep can have on hormonal balance, energy levels, and mood – all critical components for fostering a satisfying and enriching intimate life.

1. Understanding the Sleep-Sex Connection:

Delve into the intricate relationship between sleep and sexual health. Uncover the physiological and psychological mechanisms that underscore this connection, including the role of sleep in regulating hormones such as testosterone and cortisol. Gain insight into how sleep quality directly influences desire, arousal, and overall sexual satisfaction.

Practical Insight: Prioritize consistent sleep patterns by establishing a regular sleep schedule. Going to bed and waking up at the same time each day helps regulate your body's internal clock, contributing to improved sleep quality.

2. Creating a Sleep-Friendly Environment:

Explore the elements of a conducive sleep environment that promotes restful and rejuvenating sleep. From optimizing bedroom lighting and temperature to choosing comfortable bedding, discover practical tips to enhance the quality of your sleep. Uncover the importance of creating a calming bedtime routine that signals to your body that it's time to wind down.

Practical Insight: Limit exposure to screens before bedtime. The blue light emitted by devices can interfere with the production of the sleep hormone melatonin. Consider engaging in relaxing activities, such as reading a book, to prepare your mind and body for sleep.

3. Establishing Healthy Sleep Habits:

Dive into habits and practices that contribute to maintaining healthy sleep patterns. From the impact of regular exercise on sleep quality to the role of diet in promoting restful sleep, explore lifestyle choices that positively influence your ability to achieve and sustain a good night's sleep.

Practical Insight: Experiment with relaxation techniques, such as deep breathing exercises or gentle stretching, before bedtime. Incorporating these practices can help alleviate stress and tension, promoting a more relaxed and restful sleep.

As you navigate the intricate relationship between sleep and sensuality, remember that prioritizing quality sleep is an investment in your overall well-being. By incorporating these practical strategies into your routine, you not only enhance your sleep but also contribute to a more vibrant and fulfilling intimate experience.

PART IV: TARGETED SOLUTIONS FOR SPECIFIC SEXUAL HEALTH CONCERNS

As we journey deeper into understanding the nuances of sexual health, Part IV addresses specific concerns individuals may encounter, offering targeted solutions to enhance well-being and satisfaction. Each chapter focuses on distinct aspects, providing insights, guidance, and evidence-backed strategies tailored to address hormonal imbalances, stress-related intimacy issues, and fertility challenges.

9 HORMONAL IMBALANCES: DIETARY AND LIFESTYLE SOLUTIONS

Hormonal imbalances can intricately affect various aspects of sexual health, from desire to overall satisfaction. This chapter is designed to guide individuals through a comprehensive understanding of hormonal harmony and equip them with practical dietary and lifestyle solutions to restore balance and foster optimal well-being.

1. Understanding Hormonal Harmony:

Embark on a journey to comprehend the intricate dance of hormones that shape sexual health. Recognize the significance of hormonal balance in sustaining desire, arousal, and overall satisfaction. Gain insights into the interconnectedness of nutrition, lifestyle choices, and hormonal equilibrium, laying the groundwork for informed and empowered decision-making.

Practical Insight: Consider maintaining a hormonal health journal to track patterns in mood, energy, and sexual desire. This can offer valuable insights into potential imbalances and guide you towards targeted solutions.

2. Dietary Strategies for Hormonal Balance:

Unlock the transformative power of nutrition in addressing hormonal imbalances. Explore specific foods rich in essential nutrients that play a role in hormonal health. From omega-3 fatty acids to antioxidants, discover dietary strategies to support hormonal balance and enhance overall well-being.

Practical Insight: Incorporate hormone-balancing foods into your meals, such as fatty fish, flaxseeds, and colorful fruits and vegetables. These nutrient-dense choices contribute to the synthesis and regulation of key hormones.

3. Lifestyle Adjustments for Hormonal Health:

Navigate the landscape of lifestyle modifications that positively impact hormonal balance. Dive into stress management techniques that reduce cortisol levels, a hormone linked to stress. Explore the role of regular physical activity in supporting hormonal health, promoting a dynamic equilibrium for optimal functioning.

Practical Insight: Integrate mindfulness practices, such as meditation or yoga, into your daily routine. These activities not only help manage stress but also contribute to hormonal balance by promoting relaxation and overall well-being.

By understanding the intricacies of hormonal balance and implementing targeted dietary and lifestyle adjustments, individuals can take proactive steps toward enhancing their sexual health. This chapter empowers readers to make informed choices that align with their unique needs, contributing to a more harmonious and satisfying intimate life.

10 STRESS-RELATED INTIMACY ISSUES: A COMPREHENSIVE APPROACH

Stress, a ubiquitous part of modern life, can significantly impact the intimate fabric of relationships. This chapter takes a comprehensive approach to address stress-related intimacy issues, offering practical strategies to manage stress effectively and rekindle the flame of connection within relationships.

1. The Impact of Stress on Intimacy:

Dive into the profound ways stress influences intimate relationships, affecting desire, communication, and overall satisfaction. Understand the physiological responses to stress, such as elevated cortisol levels, which can contribute to decreased libido and sexual function. Recognize the interconnectedness of stress and intimacy, laying the foundation for a holistic and informed approach.

Practical Insight: Develop a shared understanding of stressors within the relationship. Open communication about individual stressors fosters empathy and strengthens the bond between partners.

2. Stress Management Techniques for Enhanced Intimacy:

Explore a diverse array of stress management techniques designed to mitigate the impact of stress on intimate well-being. From mindfulness practices to progressive muscle relaxation, discover tools that cultivate resilience and restore emotional connection. These techniques empower individuals and couples to navigate stressors collaboratively, fostering an environment conducive to intimacy.

Practical Insight: Establish a joint stress-relief ritual. This could be a daily walk together, a mindfulness session, or even a shared hobby. The act of facing stressors as a team can strengthen the emotional connection between partners.

3. Building Emotional Resilience:

Recognize the pivotal role of emotional resilience in navigating stress and rekindling intimacy. Explore strategies to fortify emotional strength, such as fostering positive communication, expressing gratitude, and creating shared goals. Building emotional resilience not only supports individuals in coping with stress but also strengthens the foundation of trust and intimacy within the relationship.

Practical Insight: Engage in activities that bring joy and laughter into the relationship. Laughter is a powerful stress-reliever and can create a positive atmosphere that enhances emotional connection.

By embracing a comprehensive approach to managing stress and cultivating emotional resilience, individuals and couples can overcome the challenges that stress poses to intimacy. This chapter serves as a guide, offering practical tools and strategies to not only weather the storms of stress but to emerge with a stronger, more connected relationship.

11 FERTILITY CHALLENGES: A ROADMAP TO CONCEPTION

1. Navigating Fertility Fitness:

Embarking on the journey to conceive starts with understanding your body's natural rhythms. Learn about menstrual cycles, ovulation, and identifying fertile windows. Use simple methods like tracking basal body temperature or ovulation prediction kits to pinpoint the best times for conception.

Practical Step: Start charting your menstrual cycle. Mark the days and observe patterns, helping you predict when you're most likely to conceive.

2. Dietary Guidance for Fertility Enhancement:

Explore how your diet can support fertility. Discover foods rich in nutrients essential for reproductive health. Include antioxidants and omega-3 fatty acids in your meals, contributing to a fertility-friendly environment.

Practical Step: Introduce fertility-boosting foods into your diet, such as leafy greens, berries, and fatty fish. Make gradual changes for a sustainable and nourishing approach.

3. Lifestyle Choices to Boost Fertility:

Make lifestyle adjustments that positively impact fertility. Maintain a healthy weight, manage stress, and avoid harmful substances. These simple changes contribute to creating an environment that supports successful conception.

Practical Step: Incorporate moderate exercise into your routine. A brisk walk or gentle yoga session can boost overall health and fertility without causing unnecessary stress.

In this chapter, we simplify the complexities of fertility challenges, offering practical steps for your journey to conception. By understanding your body, making simple dietary adjustments, and adopting fertility-friendly lifestyle choices, you empower yourself on the path to building a family. Remember, each step brings you closer to your goal, and this roadmap is designed to make the process easy to navigate.

PART V: YOUR DAILY WELLNESS CHECKLIST

As we conclude our journey through the intricacies of sexual health, Part V introduces a practical and actionable guide for daily well-being. This section provides a checklist curated to support sustainable sexual health. By incorporating these daily habits into your routine, you foster a holistic approach to well-being that goes beyond momentary fixes, promoting long-term intimate wellness.

12 DAILY WELLNESS CHECKLIST: A PRACTICAL GUIDE TO SUSTAINABLE SEXUAL HEALTH

1. Morning Rituals for a Positive Start:
• Begin your day with intention. Incorporate activities like morning stretches, deep breathing exercises, or a moment of gratitude to set a positive tone for the day. These rituals contribute to overall well-being and create a foundation for a satisfying intimate life.
Practical Step: Designate a few minutes each morning for a simple stretching routine to awaken your body and promote circulation.

2. Nutrient-Rich Meals for Vitality:
• Fuel your body with nutrient-dense meals in the course of the day. Emphasize a balanced diet rich in fruits, vegetables, lean proteins, and whole grains. These choices not only support overall health but also contribute to sustained energy levels and sexual vitality.
Practical Step: Plan your meals ahead, ensuring a colorful variety of fruits and vegetables are part of your daily intake.

3. Mindfulness Breaks for Stress Management:
• Integrate short mindfulness breaks into your day to manage stress. Whether it's a brief meditation, a mindful walk, or a moment of focused breathing, these breaks enhance emotional well-being and foster resilience in the face of daily challenges.
Practical Step: Set aside a few minutes during your workday for a mini-meditation or mindful breathing exercise

<table>
<tr><td>4. Stay Hydrated for Overall Wellness:</td></tr>
<tr><td>• Hydration is key to overall health, including sexual health. Ensure you stay well-hydrated throughout the day by drinking an adequate amount of water. Hydration supports bodily functions, including circulation and hormonal balance.</td></tr>
<tr><td>Practical Step: Carry a reusable water bottle with you as a reminder to stay hydrated, aiming for at least eight glasses of water a day.</td></tr>
</table>

<table>
<tr><td>5. Evening Routine for Relaxation:</td></tr>
<tr><td>• Wind down in the evening with a relaxation routine. Whether it's reading a book, practicing gentle stretches, or engaging in a calming activity, these practices signal to your body that it's time to transition from the day's activities to rest.</td></tr>
<tr><td>Practical Step: Create a calming bedtime routine, avoiding screens and engaging in activities that promote relaxation.</td></tr>
</table>

This checklist is a simple yet powerful guide for weaving sustainable wellness practices into your daily life. By adopting these habits, you cultivate a foundation for long-term intimate well-being, promoting a fulfilling and satisfying quality of life.

CONCLUSION

As we conclude our exploration of sexual health in "How Not to Suffer," it becomes evident that the path to a fulfilling and vibrant intimate life is multifaceted. Throughout this journey, we've uncovered the intricacies of hormonal balance, stress management, fertility, and the transformative power of nutrition and lifestyle choices.

In the pursuit of optimal sexual health, the key lies not in isolated fixes but in the integration of sustainable habits into your daily routine. By understanding the interplay of factors influencing sexual well-being and adopting practical strategies, you empower yourself to navigate challenges and cultivate a harmonious and satisfying intimate life.

This journey doesn't end with the last page of this book but extends into your daily life. The wellness checklist provided in Part V is a practical guide to reinforce these habits, promoting long-term well-being. Remember that every small step you take, whether it's embracing nutrient-rich meals, incorporating mindfulness, or fostering emotional resilience, contributes to the larger tapestry of your intimate health.

As you chart your course forward, consider this not as a conclusion but as a commencement—a commencement of a conscious and informed approach to your intimate well-being. Your journey toward sustained sexual health is a dynamic process, and with each intentional step, you pave the way for a life filled with vitality, connection, and satisfaction.

May this book serve as a companion on your ongoing journey to a thriving and fulfilling intimate life. Here's to your well-being, joy, and the vibrant tapestry of experiences that lie ahead.

Charting Your Path to Long-Term Intimate Wellness

Congratulations on reaching this section—a pivotal moment where you actively engage in mapping your journey towards long-term intimate wellness. This isn't just a conclusion but a commencement, an opportunity to chart a course that aligns with your unique needs and aspirations. Here's a practical guide to assist you in navigating this path:

1. Reflect on Your Insights:

• Take a moment to reflect on the insights gained throughout this book. Consider how hormonal balance, stress management, nutrition, and lifestyle choices intersect in your life. Identify key takeaways that resonate with you.

2. Set Personal Goals:

• Based on your reflections, set personal goals for your intimate wellness. These can be small, achievable steps that align with the principles discussed in the book. Whether it's incorporating more nutrient-rich foods, adopting stress-management techniques, or enhancing communication in your relationships, set intentions that are realistic and meaningful to you.

3. Create a Wellness Routine:

• Develop a daily wellness routine that incorporates the habits outlined in the checklist. Tailor it to your schedule and preferences, ensuring that it becomes an integral part of your day. Consistency is key in cultivating sustainable wellness practices.

4. Monitor Your Progress:

• Keep track of your progress as you implement changes into your routine. Whether it's journaling, using apps, or simply noting changes in how you feel, monitoring your journey provides valuable insights into what works best for you.

5. Seek Support and Guidance:

• Don't hesitate to seek support from healthcare professionals, nutritionists, or counselors if needed. Your journey is unique, and professionals can provide personalized guidance to enhance your intimate well-being.

6. Celebrate Achievements:
• Celebrate each small and considerable achievements alongside the way.. Recognize the positive changes in your energy levels, emotional well-being, and intimate experiences. Cultivate a positive mindset that reinforces your commitment to long-term well-being.

Remember, this is your journey, and each step you take contributes to the narrative of your intimate wellness. Embrace the process, be kind to yourself, and cherish the progress you make. As you chart your path, may it lead you to a life filled with vitality, connection, and the fulfillment of your intimate well-being.